TOM VELENCIA

Self Guide To Health & Fitness

I hope you like my book I would greatly appreciate it if you could go to Amazon and give me a rating of this book. Thank You So Much. Tom

First edition

ISBN: 9798301690969

This book was professionally typeset on Reedsy.
Find out more at reedsy.com

Table of Contents Page

Introduction

Understanding Health

Health is not merely the absence of disease but a dynamic state of complete physical, mental, and social well-being. This guide aims to empower you with the knowledge and tools to take charge of your health journey.

The Importance of a Holistic Approach

An integrated approach to health considers the entire individual. You can create a balanced and sustainable health routine by addressing physical fitness, nutrition, mental well-being, and lifestyle habits.

Chapter 1: The Foundations of Health

What Does It Mean to Be Healthy?

Explore the different dimensions of health, including physical, emotional, social, and spiritual well-being.

The Mind-Body Connection

Learn how mental health affects physical health and vice versa. Discover techniques to foster a positive mindset.

Setting Realistic Health Goals

Establish SMART (Specific, Measurable, Achievable, Relevant, Time-bound) goals to guide your health journey.

Chapter 2: Eating Healthy

Understanding Macronutrients and Micronutrients

Macronutrients: Carbohydrates, Proteins, and Fats

Micronutrients: Vitamins and Minerals

Meal Planning Basics

Learn how to plan your meals for the week, considering your nutritional needs and preferences.

Building a Balanced Plate
Discover the principles of part control and how to create balanced meals.

Healthy Snacking Ideas

Snack smartly with nutritious options that keep your energy levels stable.

The Role of Hydration

Understand the importance of water and how to ensure you are adequately hydrated.

Chapter 3: Juicing for Health

Benefits of Juicing

Discuss how juicing can enhance your nutrient intake and promote overall health.

Essential Juicing Ingredients: Explore various fruits and vegetables that are excellent for juicing.

Recipes for Health-Boosting Juices

Green Detox Juice: Spinach, cucumber, apple, lemon, ginger Immune-Boosting Citrus Juice: Orange, grapefruit, lemon, turmeric Anti-Inflammatory Beet Juice: Beetroot, carrot, apple, ginger

Tips for Getting Started with Juicing

Practical advice for incorporating juicing into your daily routine.

Chapter 4: The Anti-Inflammatory Diet

Understanding Inflammation and Its Effects

Learn how chronic inflammation can lead to various health issues.

Foods to Include in an Anti-Inflammatory Diet Emphasize the importance of whole foods, healthy fats, and spices like turmeric.

Foods to Avoid

Find common inflammatory foods such as processed sugars and trans fats.

Meal Plan for a Week of Anti-Inflammatory Eating

A sample meal plan to kick start your anti-inflammatory journey.

Chapter 5: Exercises for Every Level

The Importance of Regular Exercise

Discuss the physical and mental benefits of staying active.

Types of Exercise
Cardiovascular: Running, cycling, swimming
Strength Training: Weightlifting, body weight exercises
Flexibility and Balance: Yoga, Pilates
Creating a Balanced Workout Routine
Learn how to combine diverse types of exercises for the

best health.

routine.

Breathing Exercises and Meditation
Simple techniques to reduce stress and improve focus.

Finding Balance in a Busy World
Strategies for keeping healthy in a hectic lifestyle.

Chapter 8: Building Healthy Habits

The Science of Habit Formation
Learn how habits are formed and how to create lasting changes.

Tips for Making Lasting Changes
Practical steps to integrate healthy habits into your life.

Overcoming Obstacles and Setbacks
Strategies for dealing with challenges and staying on track.

Celebrating Your Progress
Recognize and reward your achievements, no matter how small.

Chapter 9: Putting It All Together

Creating Your Personalized Health Plan
A step-by-step guide to designing your health plan based on your goals.

Setting Goals and Milestones

Learn how to set short and long-term goals for continuous improvement.

The Importance of Community and Support
Explore the benefits of having a support system in your health journey.

Continuous Learning and Adaptation
Stay informed and be open to adjusting your health plan as needed.

Conclusion

Embracing Your Health Journey
A final note on the importance of commitment and self-love in your health journey.

Staying Informed and Inspired
Please encourage you to seek additional information and resources to continue your
growth.

Appendices
Resources for Further Reading
A curated list of books, websites, and articles on health and wellness.

Sample Shopping List
A practical shopping list to help you stock your kitchen with healthy foods.

Exercise Glossary

Definitions of standard exercise terms and concepts.

Juice Recipe Index

An index of all juice recipes is included in the book for easy reference.

Chapter 1

The Foundations of Health

What Does It Mean to Be Healthy?

Health is often defined simply as the absence of disease; however, this narrow perspective overlooks the complexity of being truly healthy. Health encompasses physical, mental, emotional, and social well-being. A holistic understanding of health acknowledges that these dimensions are interconnected and influence others.

1. Physical Health: This refers to the state of your body and its ability to perform daily activities. It includes factors such as fitness level, nutrition, and the absence of chronic illness. Physical health involves regular exercise, a balanced diet, sufficient sleep, and routine check-ups.
2. Mental Health: Mental health is equally essential and includes emotional well-being, stress management, and coping with life's challenges. It reflects how we think, feel,

and act. Good mental health enhances our ability to enjoy life and handle stress.

3. Emotional Health: This aspect focuses on understanding and managing emotions. Emotional health allows you to express feelings appropriately, cope with stress, and build healthy relationships. It is about feeling positive and enthusiastic about life.

4. Social Health: Social connections and relationships with others significantly affect overall health. Social health involves having solid and supportive relationships, engaging in social activities, and feeling connected to a community.

Understanding health as a multifaceted concept helps you appreciate that improvement in one area can lead to enhancements in others. For example, regular physical activity can boost your mood and improve your mental health, while a supportive social network can motivate you to keep a healthy lifestyle.

The Mind-Body Connection

The mind-body connection is a powerful and intricate relationship that influences overall health. This connection suggests that our thoughts, feelings, beliefs, and attitudes can affect physical health.

1. Stress and Physical Health: Chronic stress has been linked to various health issues, including heart disease, obesity, diabetes, and autoimmune disorders. Understanding how stress changes your body can help you develop effective coping strategies.

2. The Power of Positive Thinking: Research has shown

that a positive outlook on life can lead to better health outcomes. Positive thinking can enhance your immune system, reduce inflammation, and improve your overall quality of life.

3. Mindfulness and Healing: Mindfulness, meditation, and yoga can promote relaxation and reduce stress. These practices help you become more aware of your thoughts and feelings, enabling you to respond to challenges with greater resilience.

4. Emotional Expression: Suppressing emotions can negatively affect your physical health. Expressing emotions appropriately and seeking support can enhance mental and physical well-being.

Setting Realistic Health Goals

Setting goals is a vital step in your health journey. However, setting realistic, achievable goals to foster motivation and success is essential. Here are some strategies to help you set and reach your health goals:

1. SMART Goals: Use the SMART criteria to set your goals:

Specific: Could you clearly define what you want to achieve? Instead of saying, "I want to get fit," specify, "I want to exercise for 30 minutes five times a week."

Measurable: Decide how you will measure progress. For instance, track your workouts in a journal or use a fitness app.

Achievable: Because of your current situation and resources, please make sure your goals are attainable. If you're new to exercise, start with shorter workouts and gradually increase duration and intensity.

Relevant: Choose goals that matter to you and align with your health vision. If improving cardiovascular health is important, focus on activities enhancing heart health.

Time-bound: Set a deadline for your goals. This creates a sense of urgency and helps you stay accountable. For example, "I will run a 5 k event in three months."

2. Break It Down: Large goals can feel overwhelming. Break them down into smaller, manageable tasks that you can achieve daily or weekly.

3. Be Flexible: Life can be unpredictable. Be willing to adjust your goals as needed. If you meet obstacles, reassess and modify your plan rather than giving up entirely.

4. Celebrate Achievements: Acknowledge your progress along the way. Celebrating small victories boosts motivation and reinforces positive behavior changes.

5. Seek Support: Sharing your goals with friends, family, or a health coach can provide encouragement and accountability. You can join groups or communities with similar health interests for added support.

Conclusion

This chapter proves that health is a multifaceted concept encompassing physical, mental, emotional, and social well-being. The mind-body connection is crucial to overall health, emphasizing managing stress and fostering positive thoughts. Setting realistic and achievable health goals using the SMART criteria will guide you toward improved health.

As you move forward to the next chapter, remember that understanding the foundations of health is the first step in creating a fulfilling and balanced life. Embrace the journey ahead and recognize that every small step contributes to your well-being.

Chapter 2

Eating Healthy

Eating healthy is a cornerstone of overall health and well-being. It fuels our bodies, supports mental health, and plays a crucial role in disease prevention. This chapter will explore the fundamentals of healthy eating, including understanding macronutrients and micronutrients, meal planning, building a balanced diet, and smart snacking.

Understanding Macronutrients and Micronutrients

To eat healthily, it's essential to understand the different nutrients our bodies need. Nutrients can be categorized into two main groups: macronutrients and micronutrients.

Macronutrients

Macronutrients are the nutrients required in more significant amounts that provide energy and support bodily functions. They include:

1. Carbohydrates: Carbohydrates are the body's primary energy source. They can be classified into simple carbohydrates (sugars) and complex carbohydrates (starches and fiber). Aim to consume whole grains, fruits, vegetables, and legumes, which provide energy, fiber, and essential nutrients.

Sources: Brown rice, quinoa, whole-grain bread, oats, fruits, vegetables, and legumes.

2. Proteins: Proteins are essential for building and repairing tissues, making enzymes and hormones, and supporting immune function. They are made up of essential amino acids, some of which must be obtained through diet.

Sources: Lean meat, poultry, fish, eggs, dairy products, legumes, nuts, and seeds.

3. Fats: Fats are a concentrated energy source and are vital for absorbing fat-soluble vitamins (A, D, E, and K). Focus on healthy fats, such as monounsaturated and polyunsaturated fats, while limiting saturated and trans fats.

Sources: Avocados, olive oil, nuts, seeds, fatty fish, and nut butter.

Micronutrients

Micronutrients are vitamins and minerals required in smaller amounts but are crucial for various bodily functions. They support immune function, energy production, and bone health, among other roles.

1. Vitamins: These organic compounds are vital for various metabolic processes. Each vitamin has specific functions, and deficiencies can lead to health issues.

- Examples: Vitamin C (immune health), B vitamins (energy metabolism), and Vitamin D (bone health).

2. Minerals: These inorganic elements are essential for muscle contraction, nerve transmission, and fluid balance.
   - Examples: Calcium (bone health), iron (oxygen transport), and magnesium (muscle function).

Balancing Macronutrients and Micronutrients

A well-balanced diet includes a variety of foods that provide the necessary macronutrients and micronutrients. Aim for a colorful plate incorporating different food groups to ensure you get a wide range of nutrients.

Meal Planning Basics

Meal planning effectively ensures you eat healthily, save time, and reduce food waste. Here are some steps to help you get started:

1. Assess Your Needs: Consider your dietary preferences, nutritional requirements, and goals. Are you looking to lose weight, build muscle, or keep health?
2. Create a Weekly Plan: Set aside time to plan your meals. Include breakfast, lunch, dinner, and snacks. Aim for a mix of foods from all food groups.

3 Make a Grocery List: Create a shopping list based on your meal plan. Stick to the list to avoid impulse purchases of unhealthy foods.

4. Prep Ahead: Prepare meals or ingredients in advance. Batch cooking and portioning meals can make it easier to stick to your plan during busy days.

5. Stay Flexible: Life can be unpredictable. Be open to adjusting your meal plan as needed. If you find yourself with leftovers, incorporate them into your next meal.

Building a Balanced Plate

When creating balanced meals, the "balanced plate" concept can serve as a helpful guideline. Here's how to build a healthy plate:

1. Fill Half Your Plate with Fruits and Vegetables. Aim for assorted colors and types. Fresh, frozen, or canned (without added sugar or salt) options are all excellent choices.
2. Include Lean Proteins: Fill one-quarter of your plate with lean protein sources. This can include chicken, turkey, fish, beans, lentils, or tofu.
3. Add Whole Grains: The remaining quarter of your plate should consist of whole grains. Look for options like brown rice, quinoa, or whole-grain pasta.
4. Healthy Fats: Include healthy fats in moderation. This can be a drizzle of olive oil on your salad, a handful of nuts, or avocado slices.
5. Stay Hydrated: Don't forget about hydration. Aim to drink water throughout the day and consider herbal teas or infused water for variety.

Healthy Snacking Ideas

Snacking can be an excellent way to maintain energy levels and keep hunger at bay. However, it's essential to choose healthy options. Here are some nutritious snack ideas:

1. Fruits: Fresh fruits like apples, bananas, berries, and oranges are great choices. Pair them with nut butter for added protein and healthy fats.
2. Vegetables and Dip: Carrot sticks, cucumber slices, and bell pepper strips can be paired with hummus, guacamole, or yogurt-based dips.
3. Nuts and Seeds: A small handful of mixed nuts or seeds can provide healthy fats and protein. Be mindful of portion sizes, as they are calorie dense.
4. Greek Yogurt: This protein-packed snack can be enjoyed plain or topped with fresh fruit, honey, or granola for added flavor.
5. Whole Grain Snacks: Look for whole grain crackers or rice cakes, which can be paired with cheese, nut butter, or avocado.
6. Smoothies: Blend your favorite fruits and vegetables with yogurt or milk for a nutrient-dense snack. Add spinach or kale for an extra boost.

Conclusion

Eating healthy is a fundamental aspect of overall well-being. By understanding macronutrients and micronutrients, planning your meals, creating balanced plates, and choosing nutritious snacks, you can take significant steps toward improving your health.

In the next chapter, we will delve into the world of juicing and explore how it can enhance your nutrition and support your health goals. Remember that healthy eating is not about strict diets or deprivation; it's about incorporating various foods that nourish your body and make you feel good. Start small and make sustainable changes for you overall.

Chapter 3

Juicing for Health

Juicing has gained popularity as a convenient way to increase your intake of fruits and vegetables, boost your nutrient levels, and support overall health. This chapter will explore the benefits of juicing and essential juicing ingredients and provide delicious, health-boosting juice recipes.

Benefits of Juicing

Juicing can offer numerous health benefits when incorporated into a balanced diet:

1. **Nutrient Boost**: Juicing allows you to consume a concentrated source of vitamins, minerals, and antioxidants in fruits and vegetables. This can be particularly beneficial if you need help to meet your daily intake of these foods.
2. **Digestive Health**: Fresh juices are rich in enzymes and

fiber (if pulp is included), aiding digestion and improving gut health. Certain juices, mainly those high in fiber, can promote regular bowel movements.

3. **Hydration**: Juices contribute to your daily fluid intake, keeping you hydrated. Staying hydrated is vital for overall health, energy levels, and skin health.

4. **Detoxification**: Many people use juicing as part of a detox program. While the body has natural detoxification systems (primarily the liver and kidneys), juicing can support these processes by providing nutrients that help eliminate toxins.

5. **Weight Management**: Juicing can be a low-calorie, nutrient-dense choice for those seeking to lose or maintain a healthy weight. However, balancing juices with whole foods is crucial to ensure adequate protein and healthy fats.

6. **Increased Energy**: Many people feel energized after incorporating fresh juices into their diet. This may be due to the abundance of vitamins and minerals that support energy production in the body.

Essential Juicing Ingredients

About juicing, not all fruits and vegetables are created equal. Here are some essential ingredients to include in your juices for best health benefits:

1. Leafy Greens: Spinach, kale, and Swiss chard are nutrient powerhouses packed with vitamins A, C, and K and essen-

tial minerals like calcium and magnesium. They also have chlorophyll, which may aid in detoxification.

2. Fruits: Fruits like apples, oranges, pineapples, and berries add natural sweetness and a wealth of vitamins and antioxidants. Choose organic, when possible, to reduce exposure to pesticides.

3. Roots and Tubers: Beets, carrots, and ginger are excellent additions. Beets are known for their high nitrate content, which may improve blood flow and athletic performance, while ginger can aid digestion and has anti-inflammatory properties.

4. Citrus: Lemons and limes enhance flavor and are rich in vitamin C, which supports immune function and skin health.

5. Herbs: Fresh herbs like parsley, cilantro, and mint can add a refreshing flavor while providing other nutrients and antioxidants.

6. Spices: Turmeric and cinnamon can be added for their anti-inflammatory and antioxidant properties. Turmeric has curcumin, a compound known for its health benefits.

Recipes for Health-Boosting Juices

Now that you understand the benefits of juicing and the ingredients to use, here are some delicious juice recipes to get you started:

Green Detox Juice
Ingredients:
2 cups of spinach
One cucumber
One green apple

One lemon (peeled)
1-inch piece of ginger (peeled)
Water (optional for thinning)

Instructions:

1. Wash all ingredients thoroughly.
2. Cut the cucumber and apple into smaller pieces to fit into your juicer.
3. Juice all ingredients together.
4. If the juice is too thick, add water to reach your desired consistency. Serve at once.

Immune-Boosting Citrus Juice
Ingredients:
Two oranges (peeled)
One grapefruit (peeled)
One lemon (peeled)
One tablespoon honey (optional)
A pinch of cayenne pepper (optional, for a kick)

Instructions:

1. Peel and segment the oranges, grapefruit, and lemon.
2. Juice all the citrus fruits together.
3. Stir in honey and cayenne pepper if desired.
4. Serve chilled or over ice.

Anti-Inflammatory Beet Juice
Ingredients:
One medium beet (peeled and chopped)

Two carrots (peeled and chopped)
One apple (cored and chopped)
1-inch piece of ginger (peeled)
One lemon (peeled)

Instructions:

1. Prepare all ingredients by washing, peeling, and chopping as needed.
2. Juice the beet, carrots, apple, ginger, and lemon together.
3. Mix well and serve at once.

Refreshing Watermelon Mint Juice
Ingredients:
4 cups of seedless watermelon (cubed)
A handful of fresh mint leaves
Juice of 1 lime

Instructions:

1. Blend the watermelon cubes until smooth.
2. Strain the juice through a fine mesh sieve or cheesecloth to remove pulp (if desired).
3. Stir in lime juice and add mint leaves for garnish. Serve chilled.

Tropical Green Juice
Ingredients:
1 cup kale (stems removed)
1 cup of pineapple (cubed)
1/2 cucumber

One lime (peeled)

1 cup coconut water (optional)

Instructions:

1. Prepare all ingredients by washing and chopping as needed.
2. Juice the kale, pineapple, cucumber, and lime together.
3. Mix in coconut water for a tropical twist. Serve at once.

Tips for Getting Started with Juicing

1. Invest in a Good Juicer: A quality juicer will make the process easier and improve the quality of your juice. Consider a masticating juicer for better nutrient extraction.
2. Start Slowly: If you're new to juicing, incorporate one daily juice into your routine. Gradually increase the frequency as you become accustomed to it.
3. Use Fresh Ingredients: opt for fresh, organic produce when possible. The fresher the ingredients, the more nutrients your juice will keep.
4. Experiment with Flavors: Don't be afraid to mix and match different fruits and vegetables to find combinations that you enjoy. Juicing is a beautiful way to be creative in the kitchen.
5. Drink Immediately: Fresh juice is best consumed once after juicing to retain maximum nutrients. If you must store it, use an airtight container and consume it within 24 hours.
6. Incorporate Pulp: Don't discard the pulp! For added fiber and nutrients, you can use it in smoothies, soups, or baked goods.
7. Balance Your Diet: While juicing is a fantastic way to

increase nutrient intake, it should complement a diet rich in whole foods, including proteins, healthy fats, and whole grains.

Conclusion

Juicing can be a valuable addition to your health journey, offering a convenient way to boost your intake of fruits and vegetables while reaping various health benefits. With a wide array of ingredients and countless flavored combinations, you can create delicious juices that support your health goals.

As you explore the world of juicing, remember to incorporate it into a balanced diet and lifestyle. In the next chapter, we will delve into the principles of an anti-inflammatory diet, exploring how certain foods can help reduce inflammation and promote overall wellness. Embrace the vibrant colors and flavors of fresh juices and enjoy the nourishing benefits they bring to your life!

Chapter 4

The Anti-Inflammatory Diet

Chronic inflammation is increasingly recognized as a significant factor in various health conditions, including heart disease, diabetes, arthritis, and certain cancers. An anti-inflammatory diet emphasizes foods that help reduce inflammation and promote overall health. In this chapter, we will explore the concept of inflammation, foods to include and avoid and provide a sample meal plan to help you implement an anti-inflammatory diet.

Understanding Inflammation and Its Effects

What is Inflammation?

Inflammation is a natural response of the body's immune system to injury or infection. It is a protective mechanism, helping the body heal and fight pathogens. However, when inflammation becomes chronic, it can lead to numerous health issues. Chronic inflammation can result from various factors, including poor diet, stress, lack of exercise, and exposure to environmental toxins.

The Effects of Chronic Inflammation

Chronic inflammation can contribute to a range of health problems, including:

1. Heart Disease: Inflammation can lead to plaque buildup in arteries, increasing the risk of heart attacks and strokes.
2. Diabetes: Chronic inflammation is linked to insulin resistance, a key factor in type 2 diabetes development.
3. Arthritis: Inflammatory conditions, such as rheumatoid arthritis, can lead to joint pain, swelling, and stiffness.
4. Cancer: Some studies suggest that chronic inflammation may play a role in the development of certain cancers.
5. Autoimmune Disorders: Inflammation can trigger immune responses that mistakenly attack healthy tissues, leading to autoimmune diseases.

Foods to Include in an Anti-Inflammatory Diet

The anti-inflammatory diet focuses on whole, nutrient-dense foods that provide essential vitamins, minerals, and antioxidants. Here are key food groups to include:

1. Fruits and Vegetables

Fruits and vegetables are rich in vitamins, minerals, fiber, and antioxidants, which help combat inflammation. Aim for a variety of colors to maximize nutrient intake.

Berries: Blueberries, strawberries, and blackberries are

high in antioxidants called anthocyanins, which have anti-inflammatory properties.

Leafy Greens: Spinach, kale, and Swiss chard are loaded with vitamins A, C, and K, as well as anti-inflammatory compounds.

Cruciferous Vegetables: Broccoli, cauliflower, and Brussels sprouts have sulforaphane, which has been shown to reduce inflammation.

2. Healthy Fats

Healthy fats play a crucial role in reducing inflammation. Focus on sources of omega-3 fatty acids and monounsaturated fats.

Fatty Fish: Salmon, mackerel, sardines, and trout are rich in omega-3 fatty acids, which have been shown to decrease inflammation.

Olive Oil: Extra virgin olive oil is high in monounsaturated fats and has oleocanthal, a compound with anti-inflammatory properties.

Nuts and Seeds: Walnuts, chia seeds, and flax seeds provide omega-3s and antioxidants.

3. Whole Grains

Whole grains are a thorough source of fiber, which helps reduce inflammation and improve gut health.

Brown Rice: A whole grain possibility that provides essential nutrients and fiber.

Quinoa: A nutrient-dense grain that is high in protein and fiber.

Oats: Rich in beta-glucans, oats may help reduce inflammation and improve cholesterol levels.

4. Spices and Herbs

Certain spices and herbs are known for their anti-inflammatory properties and can easily be incorporated into your meals.

Turmeric: It has curcumin, a powerful anti-inflammatory compound. Adding black pepper enhances its absorption.

Ginger: Has anti-inflammatory and antioxidant effects, making it a fantastic addition to teas and dishes.

Garlic: Contains sulfur compounds that may help reduce inflammation and support immune function.

5. Legumes

Legumes, such as beans, lentils, and chickpeas, are excellent sources of protein and fiber and can help lower inflammation.

Foods to Avoid

While the anti-inflammatory diet emphasizes whole, nutrient-dense foods, it's also essential to avoid or limit certain foods that can contribute to inflammation. These include:

1. Processed Foods

Highly processed foods often have refined sugars, unhealthy fats, and additives that can trigger inflammation.

Sugary Snacks and Beverages: Candy, cookies, soda, and other sugary treats can lead to spikes in insulin and inflammation.

Processed Meats: Hot dogs, sausages, and deli meats are associated with increased inflammation and health risks.

2. Refined Carbohydrates

Refined carbohydrates can cause rapid spikes in blood sugar and insulin levels, contributing to inflammation.

White Bread and Pastries: Made with refined flour and may lack essential nutrients and fiber.

White Rice: opt for whole grains instead.

3. Trans Fats

Trans fats are unhealthy fats in many processed foods and can increase inflammation.

Fried Foods: Many fast-food items and commercially baked

goods hold trans fats.

Hydrogenated Oils: Often found in margarine and some snack foods.

4. Excessive Alcohol

While moderate alcohol consumption may have some health benefits, excessive intake can lead to inflammation and other health issues.

Meal Plan for a Week of Anti-Inflammatory Eating

To help you get started on an anti-inflammatory diet, here's a sample meal plan for one week:

Day 1

Breakfast: Overnight oats topped with blueberries, walnuts, and a drizzle of honey.

Lunch: Quinoa salad with spinach, cherry tomatoes, cucumber, and olive oil dressing.

Dinner: Grilled salmon with steamed broccoli and sweet potato.

Snack: Carrot sticks with hummus.

Day 2

Breakfast: Smoothie with spinach, banana, almond milk, and a tablespoon of flax seeds.

Lunch: Lentil soup with mixed greens and avocado.

Dinner: Stir-fried tofu with mixed vegetables (bell peppers, broccoli, carrots) and brown rice.

Snack: A handful of almonds.

Day 3

Breakfast: Greek yogurt topped with strawberries and chia seeds.

Lunch: Whole grain wrap with turkey, spinach, avocado, and tomatoes.

Dinner: Baked chicken breast with roasted Brussels sprouts and quinoa.

Snack: Sliced apple with almond butter.

Day 4

Breakfast: Chia pudding made with almond milk, topped with raspberries.

Lunch: Chickpea salad with cucumbers, parsley, and lemon dressing.

Dinner: Grilled shrimp with cauliflower rice and sauteed kale.

Snack: Celery sticks with peanut butter.

Day 5

Breakfast: Scrambled eggs with spinach and tomatoes.

Lunch: Brown rice bowl with black beans, corn, avocado, and salsa.

Dinner: Baked cod with asparagus and sweet potato wedges.

Snack: Mixed berry salad.

Day 6

Breakfast: Smoothie with kale, green apple, ginger, and lemon.

Lunch: Roasted vegetable wrap with hummus.

Dinner: Turkey chili with kidney beans and bell peppers.

Snack: Air-popped popcorn sprinkled with nutritional yeast.

Day 7

Breakfast: Oatmeal topped with sliced banana and a sprinkle of cinnamon.

Lunch: Quinoa and black bean salad with lime vinaigrette.

Dinner: Grilled vegetable skewers with brown rice.

Snack: Dark chocolate (70% cocoa or higher) with a handful of walnuts.

Conclusion

The anti-inflammatory diet emphasizes whole, nutrient-dense foods that can help reduce inflammation and promote overall health. By incorporating a variety of fruits, vegetables, healthy fats, whole grains, and spices into your meals while avoiding processed foods, refined carbohydrates, and unhealthy fats, you can take significant steps toward improving your health.

Implementing an anti-inflammatory diet can be a transformative experience, enhancing your energy levels and reducing chronic pain and disease risk. In the next chapter, we will explore exercises for every fitness level, emphasizing the importance of physical activity in keeping overall health and well-being. Embrace the power of food as medicine and enjoy the nourishing benefits of an anti-inflammatory diet!

Chapter 5

Exercises for Every Level

Regular physical activity is essential for supporting overall health and well-being. It helps manage weight, reduces the risk of chronic diseases, improves mood, and enhances quality of life. In this chapter, we will explore several types of exercise, their benefits, and how to create a balanced workout routine suitable for every fitness level.

The Importance of Regular Exercise

Regular physical activity is one of the most effective ways to promote good health. Here are some key benefits of incorporating exercise into your daily routine:

1. **Improved Cardiovascular Health**: Regular exercise strengthens the heart, improves circulation, and helps lower blood pressure and cholesterol levels.

2. **Weight Management**: Physical activity burns calories, helping them to maintain or lose weight when combined with a healthy diet.
3. **Stronger Muscles and Bones**: Weight-bearing exercises build muscle and strengthen bones, reducing the risk of osteoporosis and fractures as you age.
4. **Enhanced Mental Health**: Exercise releases endorphins, often referred to as "feel-good" hormones, which can improve mood and reduce symptoms of anxiety and depression.
5. **Increased Energy Levels**: Regular physical activity can boost your stamina and reduce feelings of fatigue.
6. **Better Sleep**: Exercise can help you fall asleep faster and enjoy deeper sleep, improving overall sleep quality.
7. **Improved Flexibility and Balance**: Activities that promote flexibility and balance can prevent injuries and enhance overall mobility.

Types of Exercise

Exercise can be categorized into several types, each with its unique benefits. Understanding these categories will help you create a well-rounded fitness routine.

1. **Cardiovascular** (Aerobic) Exercise

Cardiovascular exercise, often called aerobic exercise, increases heart and breathing rates, promoting cardiovascular health. It enhances endurance and burns calories.

Examples: Walking, running, cycling, swimming, dancing, and group fitness classes.

Recommendation: Aim for at least 150 minutes of moderate-intensity or 75 minutes of high-intensity aerobic exercise per week.

2. **Strength Training**

Strength training involves using resistance to build muscle strength and endurance. It can include free weights, resistance bands, or body weights.

Examples: Weightlifting, body weight exercises (push-ups, squats, lungs), and resistance band workouts.

Recommendation: Aim to include strength training exercises for all major muscle groups at least twice weekly.

3. **Flexibility and Stretching**

Flexibility exercises improve your range of motion and reduce the risk of injury. They can help alleviate muscle tension and promote relaxation.

Examples: Static stretching, dynamic stretching, yoga, and Pilates.

Recommendation: Incorporate flexibility and stretch exercises into your routine at least two to three times a week.

4. **Balance and Stability**

Balance exercises enhance coordination and stability, preventing falls and improving overall physical performance.

Examples: Tai chi, balance exercises (standing on one foot), and stability ball workouts.

Recommendation: Include balanced exercises in your routine, especially if you are older or at risk of falls.

Creating a Balanced Workout Routine

Creating a balanced workout routine that incorporates cardiovascular, strength, flexibility, and balance exercises is essential to achieve the best health benefits. Here's how to design your routine:

1. **Assess Your Fitness Level**

Before starting any exercise program, assess your current

fitness level. Consider your exercise experience, activity level, and health concerns or injuries.

2. **Set Realistic Goals**

Establish short-term and long-term fitness goals based on your interests and health goals. Use the SMART criteria to make your goals Specific, Measurable, Achievable, Relevant, and Time-bound.

3. **Design a Weekly Schedule**

Aim for a balanced approach that includes several types of exercise throughout the week. Here is a sample weekly workout schedule:

Sample Weekly Workout Plan:
 | Day | Activity |

Monday	30 minutes of brisk walking + 20 minutes of strength training (upper body)
Tuesday	30 minutes of cycling or swimming
Wednesday	30 minutes of strength training (lower body) + 15 minutes of stretching
Thursday	30 minutes of jogging or a dance class
Friday	20 minutes of strength training (full body) + 20 minutes of yoga
Saturday	Active rest day (light walking, gardening, or playing a sport)
Sunday	30 minutes of hiking or outdoor activity + 15 minutes of balance exercises

4. **Warm-Up and Cool Down**

Always start your workouts with a warm-up to prepare your body for exercise and reduce the risk of injury. A warm-up can include dynamic stretching or light aerobic activities for 5-10 minutes. Similarly, end your workouts with a cool-down, which may involve static stretching to help your muscles recover.

5. **Listen to Your Body**

Pay attention to how your body responds to exercise. It's normal to feel sore, especially when starting a new routine, but sharp pain or discomfort may indicate an injury. If you experience pain, stop the activity and consult a healthcare professional if necessary.

6. **Stay Motivated**

Find ways to stay motivated and make exercise enjoyable. This may include joining a fitness class, finding a workout friend, or setting challenges for yourself. Keep track of your progress and celebrate your achievements, no matter how small.

Sample Exercises for Every Level

Here are some simple exercises you can do at home or the gym, categorized by fitness level:

Beginner Level

1. Walking: A simple and effective way to begin your fitness journey. Aim for 10-15 minutes and gradually increase the duration.
2. Body weight Squats: Stand with feet shoulder-width apart, lower your body into a squat position, and return to standing. Start with 8-10 repetitions.
3. Wall Push-Ups: Stand a few feet away from a wall, place your hands on the wall, and perform push-ups by bending your elbows. Start with 5-10 repetitions.
4. Seated Leg Raises: Sit on a chair, extend one leg straight out, hold for a few seconds, and lower it. Alternate legs for 10-12 repetitions.

Intermediate Level

1. Brisk Walking or Jogging: Increase your walking pace or transition to jogging for 20-30 minutes.
2. Dumbbell Rows: With a dumbbell in each hand, bend slightly at the waist and pull the weights toward your chest. Aim for 10-15 repetitions.
3. Plank: Hold a plank position on your forearms and toes, keeping your body straight. Start with 20-30 seconds.
4. Lunges: Step forward with one leg, lowering your body until both knees are at 90-degree angles. Alternate legs for 10-12 repetitions.

Advanced Level

1. Running or Interval Training: Incorporate running or interval workouts for 30-45 minutes.
2. Dead-lifts: Using a barbell or dumbbell, stand with feet hip-width apart, hinge at the hips, and lift the weights while keeping your back straight. Aim for 8-12 repetitions.
3. Bur-pees: A full-body exercise that combines a squat, push-up, and jump. Start with 5-10 repetitions.
4. Yoga or Pilates: Join classes or follow online sessions to improve flexibility, balance, and core strength.

Conclusion

Regular exercise is vital to a healthy lifestyle, offering numerous physical and mental health benefits. By understanding the diverse types of exercise and creating a balanced workout routine tailored to your fitness level, you can achieve your health goals and enhance your well-being.

The next chapter will explore practical strategies for losing fat and building strength. Remember, the journey to better health is a marathon, not a sprint; take it one step at a time and enjoy the process!

Chapter 6

Losing Fat and Building Strength

Achieving and keeping a healthy weight while building strength involves more than just diet and exercise; it requires under-standing how your body works, setting realistic goals, and creating a sustainable plan. In this chapter, we will discuss the fundamentals of fat loss, the role of strength training, practical strategies for fat loss, and tips for tracking progress and staying motivated.

Understanding Body Composition

Before diving into fat loss and strength building, it's impor-tant to understand body composition. Body composition refers to the proportion of fat, muscle, bone, and other tissues. A healthy body composition typically involves a lower percentage of body fat and a higher percentage of lean muscle mass.

The Importance of Body Fat

While some body fat is necessary for overall health, excessive body fat can lead to numerous health risks, including:

Increased risk of chronic diseases like diabetes, heart disease, and certain cancers.

Joint issues and mobility problems.

Hormonal imbalances.

Decreased energy levels.

Conversely, building muscle mass can improve metabolism, enhance physical performance, and contribute to overall health.

Measuring Body Composition

Instead of focusing solely on weight, consider assessing your body composition through methods such as:

1. Body Fat Percentage: This can be measured through skin fold calipers, bio electrical impedance analysis, or DEXA scans.
2. Waist-to-Hip Ratio: Measure your waist and hip circumference to assess fat distribution and potential health risks.
3. Progress Photos: Regular photos can help visualize changes in body composition over time.

The Role of Strength Training in Fat Loss

Strength training is a crucial part of any fat loss program for several reasons:

1. Increased Muscle Mass: Building muscle boosts your resting metabolic rate, meaning you burn more calories at rest. This helps create a calorie deficit necessary for fat loss.
2. Enhanced Fat Oxidation: Strength training has increased

the rate at which your body burns fat for energy, especially during and after workouts.

3. Improved Body Composition: As you gain muscle and lose fat, your body composition improves, leading to a leaner physique.

4. Increased Functional Strength: Strength training enhances your ability to perform daily activities, reduces the risk of injury, and improves overall physical performance.

Effective Fat Loss Strategies

Achieving fat loss requires dietary changes, exercise, and lifestyle modifications. Here are some effective strategies to help you on your journey:

1. Create a Caloric Deficit

To lose fat, you must consume fewer calories than you spend. A safe and sustainable caloric deficit is typically around 500-1000 calories per day, which can result in a weight loss of about 1-2 pounds per week.

- Track Your Intake: Use food diaries, apps, or online tools to check your caloric intake and ensure you're meeting your goals.

2. Focus on Whole Foods

Prioritize whole, minimally processed foods that are nutrient-dense and lower in calories. This includes:

Fruits and vegetables: High in fiber and low in calories.

Lean proteins: These include chicken, turkey, fish, beans, and legumes, which promote satiety.

Whole grains: Such as brown rice, quinoa, and oats, which provide sustained energy.

3. Incorporate Strength Training

Aim to include strength training at least 2–3 times per week, focusing on all major muscle groups. Here are a few practical strength training exercises:

Squats
Dead lifts
Push-ups
Rows
Lunges

4. Include High-Intensity Interval Training (HIIT)

HIIT involves alternating between short bursts of intense exercise and rest periods or lower-intensity exercise. This method can help you burn more calories in less time and has been shown to improve fat loss.

Example HIIT Workout: 30 seconds of sprinting followed by 1 minute of walking, repeated for 15–20 minutes.

5. Stay Hydrated

Drinking enough water is essential for overall health and can aid in weight loss. Sometimes, thirst is mistaken for hunger. Aim for at least 8 cups (64 ounces) of water daily, adjusting for activity level and climate.

6. Get Enough Sleep

Sleep plays a crucial role in weight management and fat loss. Poor sleep can lead to hormonal imbalances that increase hunger and cravings. Aim for 7–9 hours of quality sleep per night.

7. Manage Stress

Chronic stress can negatively affect your ability to lose fat.

High stress levels can lead to overeating, especially high-calorie comfort foods. Practice stress management techniques such as mindfulness, meditation, yoga, or deep breathing exercises.

Tracking Progress and Staying Motivated

Tracking your progress and keeping motivation are critical components of any successful fat loss journey. Here are some tips:

1. Set SMART Goals

Establish Specific, Measurable, Achievable, Relevant, and Time-bound goals. For example, "I want to lose 2 pounds per week for the next month" is a SMART goal.

2. Keep a Journal

Document your food intake, workouts, and feelings. This can help find patterns, areas for improvement, and successes along the way.

3. Celebrating Non-Scale Victories

Focus on achievements beyond the scale, such as increased energy levels, improved endurance, fitting into smaller clothing sizes, or lifting heavier weights.

4. Finding Accountability

Share your goals with friends or join a support group or fitness class. Having accountability can help keep you motivated and on track.

5. Being Patient and Kind to Yourself

Fat loss and strength building take time. Being patient with the process and recognizing that ups and downs are normal is essential. If you experience setbacks, don't be discouraged— focus on getting back on track.

6. Mix Up Your Routine

Try new exercises, classes, or sports to keep your workout

fresh and exciting. This can prevent boredom and keep motivation.

Conclusion

Losing fat and building strength is a journey that requires a combination of a well-balanced diet, regular exercise, and lifestyle adjustments. You can achieve your health and fitness goals by understanding body composition, incorporating strength training, and using effective strategies.

In the next chapter, we will explore the connection between mindfulness, mental health, and stress management and how to cultivate a healthy mindset to support your overall well-being. Remember, every small step you take contributes to your progress; embrace the journey and celebrate your successes!

Chapter 7

Mindfulness and Stress

Management

In today's fast-paced world, managing stress and cultivating mindfulness have become increasingly crucial for keeping over-all health and well-being. Chronic stress can negatively affect physical health, mental clarity, and emotional stability. In this chapter, we will explore the impact of stress on health, techniques for fostering mindfulness, and practical strategies for effective stress management.

The Impact of Stress on Health

Stress is a natural response to challenging situations; however, when it becomes chronic, it can lead to various health issues:

1. Physical Health Problems: Chronic stress has been linked

to a range of health conditions, including heart disease, high blood pressure, obesity, diabetes, and gastrointestinal issues. Stress can trigger the release of hormones like cortisol, leading to weight gain, particularly around the abdomen.

2. Mental Health Issues: Prolonged stress can contribute to anxiety, depression, and other mental health disorders. It can impair cognitive function, leading to difficulty concentrating, memory problems, and decreased productivity.

3. Weakened Immune System: Chronic stress can weaken the immune system, making you more susceptible to infections and illnesses.

4. Sleep Disturbances: Stress often disrupts sleep patterns, leading to insomnia or poor-quality sleep. Lack of sleep can worsen stress and create a vicious cycle.

5. Emotional Strain: High stress levels can lead to irritability, mood swings, and difficulty managing emotions, affecting relationships and overall quality of life.

Mindfulness Techniques for Everyday Life

Mindfulness is fully present in the moment, seeing thoughts and feelings without judgment. It helps cultivate awareness, reduce stress, improve emotional regulation, and enhance overall well-being. Here are some mindfulness techniques to incorporate into your daily routine:

1. **Mindful Breathing**

Mindful breathing involves focusing your attention on your breath. It can be practiced anywhere and is an effective way to calm the mind.

How to Practice:

Find a quiet space and sit comfortably.

Close your eyes and take a deep breath through your nose, allowing your belly to expand.

Exhale slowly through your mouth, releasing any tension.

Continue to breathe deeply, focusing on the sensation of your breath entering and leaving your body.

If your mind wanders, gently bring your focus back to your breath.

2. Body Scan

A body scan is a mindfulness exercise that promotes awareness of physical sensations and helps release tension.

How to Practice:

Lie down or sit comfortably. Close your eyes.

Take a few deep breaths to relax.

Starting from your toes, mentally scan your body, paying attention to any sensations, tension, or discomfort.

Gradually move up through your body (feet, legs, torso, arms, neck, and head), observing how each area feels.

Acknowledge any tension and consciously relax those areas as you breathe out.

3. Mindful Eating

Mindful eating involves paying full attention to the eating experience, savoring each bite, and recognizing hunger and satiety cues.

How to Practice:

- Choose a meal or snack and drop distractions (like TV or phones).

Before eating, take a moment to see the food's colors, textures, and smells.

Take small bites, chew slowly, and savor the flavors.

Notice how your body feels as you eat and stop when you feel satisfied rather than overly full.

4. Meditation

Meditation is a structured practice that can help cultivate mindfulness and reduce stress.

How to Practice:

Set aside a specific time each day (even if just for 5-10 minutes) for meditation.

Find a quiet, comfortable space to sit or lie down.

Focus on your breath, a mantra, or guided meditation (available through apps like Head space or Calm).

If your mind wanders, gently bring your focus back to your chosen point of concentration.

5. Gratitude Journaling

Practicing gratitude can shift your focus from stressors to positive aspects of your life.

How to Practice:

Write down three things you are grateful for at the end of each day.

Reflect on why these things are meaningful and how they contribute to your well-being.

Reviewing your gratitude list regularly can help foster a positive mindset.

Finding Balance in a Busy World

Finding balance in a hectic lifestyle can be challenging, but prioritizing self-care and incorporating mindfulness can significantly enhance your overall well-being.

1. Schedule Downtime

Make time for relaxation and self-care in your daily schedule. Whether reading a book, walking, or enjoying a warm bath, prioritizing activities promotes relaxation and joy.

2. Set Boundaries

Learn to say no to commitments that overwhelm you. Establishing boundaries helps manage your time and energy, allowing you to focus on what truly matters.

3. Practice Time Management

Organize your tasks and responsibilities to reduce stress. Utilize techniques such as the Pomodoro Technique (working in focused bursts with breaks) or create a daily to-do list to enhance productivity.

4. Stay Connected

Maintain social connections with friends and family. Sharing your thoughts and feelings with others can provide support and reduce stress. Engage in social activities that bring joy and fulfillment.

5. Incorporate Movement

Physical activity is a powerful stress reliever. Incorporate regular exercise into your routine through walking, yoga, dancing, or any activity you enjoy. Exercise releases endorphins, which can improve mood and reduce stress.

6. Limit Screen Time

Excessive screen time, especially on social media, can contribute to stress and anxiety. Set boundaries on your device usage and take breaks from screens to engage in other activities.

Conclusion

Mindfulness and stress management are essential components of a balanced lifestyle. Incorporating mindfulness techniques into your daily routine and adopting practical stress management strategies can enhance your mental and emotional well-being, improve resilience, and navigate life's challenges more effectively.

The next chapter will explore how to build healthy habits that support your health and fitness goals. Remember, cultivating mindfulness is a journey—be patient with yourself and embrace the process of being present in each moment. With consistent practice, you can create a more peaceful and fulfilling life.

Chapter 8

Building Healthy Habits

Healthy habits are vital to achieving and sustaining your health and fitness goals. While motivation can spur initial changes, the development of consistent habits ultimately leads to long-term success. In this chapter, we will explore the science of habit formation, tips for making lasting changes, strategies for overcoming obstacles, and the importance of celebrating progress.

The Science of Habit Formation

Understanding how habits are formed can empower you to create positive changes in your life. Habits are routines or behaviors that become automatic over time, often triggered by specific cues or contexts. The process of habit formation can be broken down into three main components:

   1. **Cue**

A cue is a trigger that starts the habit. It can be an external signal, such as a time of day, location, or specific action, or an internal signal, such as an emotion or thought. Finding cues associated with your current habits can help you understand what prompts your behavior.

2. Routine

The routine is the behavior or action that follows the cue. This is the habit, whether exercising, eating a healthy meal, or engaging in mindfulness practices.

3. Reward

The reward is the positive outcome or benefit you receive from completing the routine. Rewards reinforce the behavior, making you more likely to repeat the habit. Understanding what motivates you can help you design effective rewards that encourage habit formation.

The Habit Loop

The habit loop consists of the cue, routine, and reward, creating a cycle reinforcing the habit. You can create new, healthier habits or break undesired ones by manipulating this loop. For example, if you want to develop a habit of exercising regularly, you might:

Cue: Set a specific time in your calendar for exercise.

Routine: Engage in your chosen workout at that time.

Reward: Treat yourself to a healthy smoothie or enjoy a relaxing bath afterward.

Tips for Making Lasting Changes

Building healthy habits takes time and effort, but you can create lasting change with the right strategies. Here are some practical tips to help you along the way:

1. **Start Small**

Begin with small, manageable changes rather than drastic overhauls. This makes it easier to adopt new habits and reduces the likelihood of feeling overwhelmed. For example, commit to a 10-minute walk each day instead of aiming for a full hour.

2. **Be Specific**

Instead of vague goals like "exercise more," set specific and measurable goals, such as "I will go for a 30-minute walk every evening after dinner." Specificity helps to clarify your intentions and makes it easier to track progress.

3. **Create a Routine**

Incorporate your new habits into your daily routine, making them part of your lifestyle. Consistency is vital; a regular schedule will help reinforce the behavior.

4. **Use Reminders**

Set reminders to prompt your new habits. You can use alarms on your phone, sticky notes in visible places, or apps that help you track your progress. Visual cues can serve as powerful motivators.

5. **Finding Accountability**

Share your goals with friends or family or consider joining a support group. Having someone to hold you accountable can provide motivation and encouragement when needed.

6. **Track Your Progress**

Keeping a journal or using a habit-tracking app can help you check your progress and stay motivated. Seeing your achievements over time can reinforce positive behavior and encourage you to keep going.

7. **Be Patient**

Habits take time to form. Research suggests that establishing a new habit can take anywhere from 21 to 66 days. Be patient with yourself and understand that setbacks are a normal part of the process. Focus on progress rather than perfection.

Overcoming Obstacles and Setbacks

Challenges and setbacks are inevitable on the journey to building healthy habits. Here are some strategies to help you navigate obstacles:

1. **Find Barriers**

Reflect on the obstacles that may hinder your progress. Common barriers include time constraints, lack of motivation, and environmental factors. Naming these barriers allows you to develop strategies to overcome them.

2. **Develop Critical Thinking Skills**

When faced with challenges, I practice critical thinking skills to find solutions. For instance, if you struggle to exercise, explore options for shorter workouts or consider incorporating activity into your daily routine (e.g., taking the stairs instead of the elevator).

3. **Stay Flexible**

Be open to adjusting your approach if something isn't working. Flexibility is essential for navigating the difficulties of habit formation. If your initial plan isn't sustainable, consider modifying it to fit your lifestyle better.

4. **Practice Self-Compassion**

Be kind to yourself when setbacks occur. Instead of being critical, practice self-compassion and recognize that everyone faces challenges. Focus on what you can learn from the experience and how to move forward.

5. Reassess Your Goals

If your goals are too ambitious or unrealistic, take a step back and reassess them. Adjusting your goals to be more achievable can help you regain motivation and confidence.

Celebrating Your Progress

Recognizing and celebrating your achievements, no matter how small, is vital for keeping motivation and reinforcing positive behavior. Here are some ways to celebrate your progress:

1. Acknowledge Achievements

Take time to reflect on your accomplishments. Whether you've successfully exercised regularly, eaten more fruits and vegetables, or reduced stress through mindfulness, acknowledging your achievements reinforces your commitment to healthy habits.

2. Treat Yourself

Reward yourself for reaching milestones. This could be simple, like eating a favorite healthy meal or enjoying a relaxing day off. Choose rewards that align with your health goals.

3. Share Your Success

Share your achievements with friends, family, or social media communities. Celebrating with others can inspire and motivate them while reinforcing your commitment to healthy habits.

4. Create a Vision Board

Visualize your goals by creating a vision board for your aspirations and achievements. Display it in a prominent place to constantly remind you what you are working toward.

Conclusion

Building healthy habits is a journey that requires time, patience, and dedication. By understanding the science of habit formation, employing effective strategies, overcoming obstacles, and celebrating your progress, you can create sustainable changes that improve health and well-being.

The next chapter will explore how to combine everything to create your personalized health plan. Remember, every small step you take brings you closer to your goals. Embrace the process, stay committed, and enjoy the journey toward a healthier you!

Chapter 9

Putting It All Together

Creating a personalized health plan is the culmination of your journey through the various aspects of health, nutrition, exercise, mindfulness, and habit formation discussed in the earlier chapters. A well-structured health plan serves as a road map that guides you toward your goals, ensuring that you incorporate the knowledge and skills you've developed. This chapter will outline how to create your personalized health plan, set goals and milestones, emphasize the importance of community and support, and encourage continuous learning and adaptation.

Creating Your Personalized Health Plan

A personalized health plan is a tailored strategy that reflects your unique goals, lifestyle, preferences, and needs. Here's how to create one:

1. **Assess Your Current Health Status**

Start by evaluating your current health and fitness levels. Consider factors such as:

Body composition (weight, body fat percentage, muscle mass)

Fitness level (cardiovascular endurance, strength, flexibility)

Dietary habits (nutritional intake, eating patterns)

Mental and emotional well-being (stress levels, sleep quality)

You can use health assessments, fitness tests, or consultations with healthcare professionals to gather this information.

2. **Define Your Goals**

Set specific, measurable, achievable, relevant, and time-bound (SMART) goals based on your assessment. Consider both short-term and long-term goals:

Short-term goals: These goals can be achieved within a few weeks or months. For example, "I will exercise for 30 minutes five times a week for the next month."

- Long-term goals: These are broader aims that may take several months or even years to achieve. For instance, "I aim to lose 20 pounds over the next six months" or "I want to run a 5 K in under 30 minutes within a year."

3. **Develop an Action Plan**

Create a detailed action plan outlining the specific steps you will take to achieve your goals. This plan should include the following:

Nutrition: Outline your dietary preferences, meal planning strategies, and specific dietary guidelines (e.g., anti-inflammatory diet, part control). Consider incorporating more whole foods, fruits, vegetables, lean proteins, and healthy fats into your meals.

Exercise: Develop a weekly workout schedule that includes cardiovascular, strength, flexibility, and balance training. Tailor the intensity, duration, and type of exercise to fit your current fitness level and goals.

Mindfulness and Stress Management: Incorporate mindfulness practices, such as meditation or mindful breathing, into your daily routine. Set aside time for relaxation and self-care to reduce stress levels.

Habit Formation: Find specific habits you want to build, such as drinking more water, getting enough sleep, or practicing gratitude. Use the strategies discussed in Chapter 8 to help set up these habits.

4. Set a Timeline

Establish a timeline for your goals and action plan. Break down your long-term goals into smaller milestones and set deadlines for each. This will help you stay on track and provide a sense of accomplishment as you reach each milestone.

5. Monitor Progress

Regularly assess your progress toward your goals. Schedule check-ins (weekly or monthly) to evaluate what's working and what may need adjustment. Use journals, apps, or fitness trackers to record your achievements and challenges.

Setting Goals and Milestones

Setting goals and milestones is crucial for keeping motivation and ensuring accountability. Here's how to effectively set and track your goals:

1. Write Down Your Goals

Putting your goals into writing solidifies your commitment. Keep your goals visible on a vision board, a planner, or a digital document. This serves as a reminder of what you are working toward.

2. Celebrating Milestones

Acknowledge and celebrate your achievements along the way. Celebrating milestones not only boosts motivation but also reinforces positive behavior. Treat yourself to a reward that aligns with your health goals, such as new workout gear, a massage, or a fun outing.

3. Adjust Goals as Needed

Life is dynamic, and circumstances may change. Be open to reassessing and adjusting your goals, as necessary. If you meet setbacks or discover an irrelevant goal, change it to fit your current situation better.

The Importance of Community and Support

Having a support system is vital for achieving your health goals. Connecting with similar aspirations can provide motivation, encouragement, and accountability. Here are some ways to build a supportive community:

1. Join a Fitness Class or Group

Participating in group fitness classes, running clubs, or sports teams can foster a sense of camaraderie and motivation. Exercising with others creates accountability and makes workouts more enjoyable.

2. Seeking Support from Friends and Family

Share your goals with friends and family members who can offer encouragement and support. Having someone to join you on your health journey can make a significant difference.

3. Use Online Communities

Consider joining online forums, social media groups, or health and wellness apps focusing on your interests. These platforms can provide resources, tips, and a sense of community.

4. Work with Professionals

If you need added guidance, consider working with health professionals such as registered dietitians, personal trainers, or health coaches. They can give personalized advice and support tailored to your needs.

Continuous Learning and Adaptation

Health and wellness are a lifelong journey that requires ongoing learning and adaptation. Stay curious and open-minded as you explore added information and strategies:

1. Stay Informed

Keep updated with the latest research, trends, and best practices in health and wellness. Read books, attend workshops, and follow reputable blogs or podcasts.

2. Experiment and Adapt

Be willing to try innovative approaches and experiment with different dietary practices, workout routines, and mindfulness techniques. What works for one person may not work for another, so find what resonates with you.

3. Reflect on Your Journey

Regularly reflect on your health journey, assessing your successes and challenges. Consider journalism or meditating to process your thoughts and feelings about your progress.

Conclusion

Creating a personalized health plan is an empowering step toward achieving your health and fitness goals. You can cultivate lasting changes in your life by assessing your current health status, defining your goals, developing an action plan, and embracing community support.

Remember that health is not a destination but a lifelong journey of growth and learning. As you implement your plan, stay patient and kind to yourself. Celebrate your progress, adapt as needed, and embrace the process of becoming the best version of yourself.

In this book, we've covered a comprehensive range of topics to support your health journey. As you move forward, keep the principles of nutrition, exercise, mindfulness, and habit-building in mind. You have the tools you need to thrive; now is the time to act and enjoy the vibrant, healthy life you deserve!

Good Luck in the Future, I hope you enjoyed this book as much as I did writing it. If you did please go to Amazon and give me a rating. Thank You. Tom

Resources

This section provides a curated list of books, websites, podcasts, and other resources to help you continue your journey toward better health and well-being. These resources cover assorted topics, including nutrition, exercise, mindfulness, and habit formation.

Books

1. Nutrition and Healthy Eating

"How Not to Die" by Michael Greger, M.D.

A comprehensive guide on how diet can prevent and reverse disease, featuring practical advice and science-backed recommendations.

"The Blue Zones Solution" by Dan Buettner

Explores the eating habits and lifestyle choices of the world's longest-lived people, offering insights into nutrition and longevity.

2. Exercise and Fitness

"The New Rules of Lifting" by Lou Schuler and Alwyn Cosgrove

A practical guide to strength training featuring comprehensive workout plans and nutritional advice.

"Yoga Anatomy" by Leslie Kaminoff and Amy Matthews

A detailed look at yoga poses' anatomy is suitable for beginners and experienced practitioners alike.

3. Mindfulness and Stress Management

"The Miracle of Mindfulness" by Thich Nhat Hanh

A guide to mindfulness practices, emphasizing the importance of being present in everyday life.

"The Power of Now" by Eckhart Tolle

An exploration of living in the present moment and freeing oneself from the burdens of past and future anxieties.

4. Habit Formation

"Atomic Habits" by James Clear

A practical guide to building good habits and breaking bad ones, emphasizing the power of tiny changes over time.

"The Power of Habit" by Charles Duhigg

An exploration of the science behind habit formation and how to create lasting change in your life.

Websites

1. Nutrition and Health

ChooseMyPlate.gov (https://www.choosemyplate.gov)

A resource from the USDA guides dietary choices and meal planning.

Nutrition.gov (https://www.nutrition.gov)

A comprehensive source of information on nutrition, dietary guidelines, and healthy eating.

2. Fitness and Exercise

American Council on Exercise (ACE) (https://www.acefitness.

<u>org</u>)

A trusted fitness and exercise information source, including workout plans and certification programs.

Fitness Blender (<u>https://www.fitnessblender.com</u>)

A website offering free workout videos and resources for all fitness levels.

3. Mindfulness and Mental Health

<u>Mindful.org</u> (<u>https://www.mindful.org</u>)

A resource for articles, practices, and courses on mindfulness and meditation.

Headspace (<u>https://www.headspace.com</u>)

A popular app for guided meditation and mindfulness practices.

Podcasts

1. Nutrition and Health

"The Model Health Show" with Shawn Stevenson

A podcast covering nutrition, fitness, and health with expert guests and practical tips.

"FoundMyFitness" with Dr. Rhonda Patrick

Focuses on health, nutrition, and the science of aging, featuring interviews with leading researchers.

2. Mindfulness and Personal Development

"The Mindfulness Meditation Podcast" by The Rubin Museum

Offers guided meditations and discussions on mindfulness practices.

"The Tony Robbins Podcast"

Covers a wide range of topics, including personal development, health, and wellness, featuring expert interviews and actionable advice.

Online Courses and Apps

1. Online Courses

Coursera (https://www.coursera.org)

Offers various nutrition, exercise science, mindfulness, and wellness courses from leading universities and institutions.

Udemy (https://www.udemy.com)

Features courses on fitness, nutrition, and mindfulness practices, allowing you to learn at your own pace.

2. Health and Fitness Apps

MyFitnessPal

A food diary app that helps you track your nutrition and exercise, making it easier to achieve your health goals.

Calm

An app focused on mindfulness and meditation, offering guided sessions and sleep stories to promote relaxation.

Conclusion

These resources serve as valuable tools to support your health journey. Exploring literature, engaging with online content, and connecting with communities can deepen your understanding of health and wellness while finding inspiration and motivation to continue making positive changes in your life. Remember that the journey to better health is ongoing; there is always more to learn and discover!